Assault in Hospitals:
Theory, Policy and Management
Your 5th Psychiatric Consultation
By William R. Yee M.D., J.D.
Copyright Applied for Aug 19, 1983

Assaults in hospitals have significant impact on patients, staff and community.[1] Assaults are often followed by notorious publicity[2] which motivates rigorous attention at intervention, prediction, preventing, training of personnel and community relations. Regulatory agencies promulgate rather detailed rules that define the conduct of hospitals and medical personnel.[3] Hospitals establish additional rules and policies in relation to aggressive and potentially homicidal patients.[4]

Assault is a derivative of human aggression. It is best understood in the content of both group and individual activity. Group activity is most often characterized as war and insurrection. Between 1820 and 1945, 60 million deaths occurred as a direct result of conflicts between groups. Since 1945, Korea, Vietnam and 500 other revolutions have added to this staggering accumulation of casualties. Group aggression continues as a significant cause of mortality and morbidity.[5]

A wide variety of motivations manifest as aggression and assault. Predatory activity, fear, irritability, territorial imperative, maternal instincts, sexual drive, male dominance and instrumental behavior all manifest with aggression and assault.[6]

Each of these categories of aggressive behavior have been studied by scientists and tested by the courts in criminal prosecution.

Predatory behavior manifests in its purest form as cannibalism. Cannibalism is manifest in Western Culture only under extreme circumstances. Criminal prosecution for cannibalism has been recorded for acts precipitated by starvation on lifeboats drifting and lost on the open seas.[7]

Fear induces self-defense. Self-defense is as well known in criminal law as in biological research.[8]

Irritable aggression is a diffuse discharge of physical activity in response to minimal stimuli. Frustration and temper tantrums are well known in Western Culture. Irritable aggression generates legal arguments regarding malice, chance-medley, provocation, recklessness, and negligence.[9]

Territorial aggression relates to the need for a minimal amount of space or a zone of privacy around each individual. Legal arguments explore the right to defend property and the need to retreat from assault to avoid the use of deadly force and homicide.[10]

Maternal aggression protects offspring and insures the survival of the biological species. Legal arguments vindicate maternal instincts and the right to utilize aggression and assault to the protection of others.[11]

Sexual homicide is a product of male competition for females or sexual foreplay and sexual arousal. Legal arguments justify or mitigate sexual aggression due to provocation, adultery, and the prevention of adultery.[12]

Intermale aggression relates to sexual, social, and territorial functions and might be described as status or macho displays between males. Legal arguments explore the motivation for aggression in mitigation of chance-medley, recklessness, and negligence.[13]

Instrumental aggression is learned and may be characterized as military, gang, or antisocial aggression according to the context. This aggression creates prosecution for conspiracy to commit homicide and aiding and abetting homicide.[14]

The United States provides a display of a very aggressive culture. Violent death is the leading cause of death between the ages of 1 and 39 and the third cause of death for all ages.[15] The total loss of expected life is greater than from any other cause of death.[16] Considering the pervasiveness of aggression in the United States, it is predictable that assault will occur any time two people associate.

Although assault is a predictable consequence of human association, it is not predictable on the basis of individual or discrete events. It is noted that emergency visits in hospitals are not determined by the nature of the psychiatric diagnosis. Symptoms such as hostility, violence and impaired judgment that create behavioral management problems and occur across the continuum of psychiatric diagnosis motivate emergency room visits and psychiatric admissions.[17]

Emergency admissions to psychiatric units are most likely to be attributable to an assessment by the admitting physician that the patient is dangerous. This is a curious finding as the weight of psychiatric literature and opinion supports the notion that prediction of dangerousness is extremely inaccurate.[19]

A flip of the coin is more accurate.[20]

Routinely finding all such patients not dangerous would result in 89% accuracy.[21]

Mental health personnel consistently over predict dangerousness to avoid strong negative public reaction to error.[22] Apparently, it is better to commit 89% harmless or less than dangerous to avoid allowing the 11% dangerous concealed within this group to roam free at large to maim and kill.

Although it is a moral, medical, and legal goal to improve prediction of dangerousness, the literature reveals little recent meaningful progress.

This is a product of many factors.

At this time the legal definition of dangerous varies from state to state.[23] Data is difficult to compare among the states.

The definition of dangerousness is not uniform. The definition of dangerousness should be made explicit prior to prediction.[24]

There should be a clear distinction between assaults that manifest as a product of normal behavior, criminal behavior, and mental illness.

Authority argues that many assaults resulting in treatment at psychiatric hospitals properly are the object of criminal prosecution rather than psychiatric intervention.[25]

Assault may be a product of either organic or psychologically derived mental illness. Organic causes of mental illness include drugs, metabolic disorders, infections, deterioration associated with age, brain tumors, genetic abnormalities, and epilepsy.

Reactions to drugs are very common causes of psychosis and aggressive behavior. Alcohol[26] and phencyclidine[27] are the most notorious drugs associated with aggression.

Epilepsy, particularly psychomotor epilepsy, has generated assaultive behavior.[28]

Genetic abnormality may produce aggressive heavier. The XYY syndrome, a chromosomal abnormality, has been known to be excessively common in prison populations.[29]

Biochemical distinctions between children with socialized and unsocialized conduct disorders have been noted.[30]

Aggression, suicide, and spinal fluid metabolism have been studied.[31]

There is considerable overlap in the criminal, psychiatric and normal populations in relation to the factor of aggression.[32]

There are a number of contributing factors. First, aggression may be a product of normal conduct[33], criminal conduct[34], or psychiatric illness[35].

Second, the criminal notion of, "mens rea," (the criminal mind) allows for a concurrent mental illness.[36]

Mental illness and mens rea are not mutually exclusive constructs.

This is most obvious in the psychiatric diagnosis of antisocial character disorder.

The criminal justice system does not allow for a diagnosis of antisocial personality as a defense.[37]

In fact, the notion of the habitual offender requires more severe penalty in states that have recidivist statutes.[38]

Psychiatrists focus on the inability to conform behavior for purposes of rehabilitation, although psychiatric intervention is admittedly ineffective.

The criminal justice system focuses on detention to protect the general population.[39] At this time about one to three percent of the population are diagnosable as antisocial personalities.

About twenty percent of the prison population is diagnosable as having an antisocial personality.[40]

There is a great deal of literature regarding the overlap of criminal and psychiatric populations. It is noted that only 0.2% of the criminal cases in the federal system result in the verdict of "not guilty by reason of insanity."[41]

However, between 15% and 20% of the prison population have psychiatric problems sufficient to justify psychiatric intervention.[42]

Observers have noted the diversion of the mentally ill into the criminal system.[43] Psychomotor epilepsy has been noted to be unusually common among violent incarcerated adolescents.[44] Drug abuse has been associated with criminal behavior among adolescents.[45] Detention and re-arrest rates have been found to be similar between convicted felons and those found not guilty by reason of insanity.[46] Finally, violent (assaultive) and suicidal behavior has been noted to be characteristic of certain groups of psychiatric patients.[47]

Whether the aggressive conduct is predictable

or unpredictable, the hospital and attending psychiatrist must manage the patient to minimize harm to other patients, staff and visitors. This duty is present whether the aggression is a product of normal behavior, criminal conduct, or mental illness. This duty has been codified in the Michigan Mental Health Code and the Rules and Regulations of the Department of Mental Health.

Interventions include interrupting the active assault and predicting potential assaults for the purpose of prevention. Interruption of an assault requires adequate personnel who are properly trained. The greater the number of personnel intervening the less likely there is to be injury.[48] The security force should remain in the area until the patient is adequately sedated or restrained.[49] Generally one should not encroach upon a patient until enough assistance is available. Minimally, one person for each limb, with extra people, the more the better, should be available.[50]

After the assault is interrupted, it is often necessary to sedate the patient. Minor tranquilizers such as diazepam (Valium) and major tranquilizers such as haloperidol have been used effectively i.m. (intramuscularly) or i.v. (intravenously).[51] Five milligrams of valium i.m. should be sufficient for the mildly obstreperous patient. Haldol is effective for unmanageable patients, the i.m. route being useful if the patient is unwilling or unable to swallow a pill. Haldol has been used i.v., although this use is not indicated by the package insert or the Physician's Desk Reference.[52] Forty to sixty milligrams have been injected i.v. over periods of time to effectively manage acute agitation manifesting with assaultive behavior.[53]

It is important to distinguish between the psychotic and nonpsychotic patient who is violent.[54] An armed psychotic patient should be disarmed by trained law enforcement personnel, as he does not respond to rational intercessions.[55]

If unarmed, the patient should be approached with overwhelming force so that there is no contest.[56]

"The violent struggling patient is most effectively subdued with an appropriate intravenous sedative, such as sodium amobarbital (Amytal sodium), 0.5 gm. Given slowly intravenously. It is most important to give intravenous medication with great care. In the excitement of the moment, there may be a tendency to inject too swiftly, with respiratory arrest and even death as a possible result.[57]"

"Better than all parental medication, is the use of electroconvulsive therapy (ECT) to control psychotic violence if this treatment modality is available on an emergency basis. The administration of a second ECT treatment 5 minutes after the first and a third ECT treatment 1 hour later usually ends an episode of psychotic violence."[58]

"Violent psychotic patients are sometimes placed into mechanical restraints. The danger of this procedure should be noted. Not only does it create a vicious cycle by intensifying the patient's psychotic terror, but, if prolonged, mechanical restraints can cause hyperthermia and in some instances of catatonic excitement, it can cause death."[59]

"Traditionally legal and psychiatric theories of dangerousness have focused upon the individual as the source of these behaviors.

More recently, a view has been emerging which focuses upon the interaction of a person with his physical and social environment in the production of behavior considered dangerous."[60]

The American Psychiatric Association (hereinafter APA) has suggested "elopsychiatry" as the designation for person-environment interactions in general.[61] The APA accepts the notion that the environment includes the biological, and physical levels all the way up to the psychosocial levels. Controversy focuses on the relative weights of individual traits as opposed to situational factors in determining behavior and clinical response to treatment.[62]

This notion is exemplified by the battered wife syndrome. One can intuitively grasp why battered children stay with their parents. Why a battered wife stays with her abusive husband is more difficult to understand.[63]

The notion of "victim mediated homicide" is startling to the average person. However, research has revealed that suicide, homicide, and accidental death are often indistinguishable, justifying the unitary notion of violent death.[64]

"In family violence, one should take note of the special vulnerability of selected close relatives. A wife or husband may have a curious masochistic attachment to the spouse in which violence is provoked by taunting and otherwise undermining the self-esteem of the partner. Such relationships commonly end in the murder of the provoking partner and sometimes in the suicide of the other."[65]

The author recommends a show of force with reassurance as the best intervention with this type of marital discord.[66]

"Milieu Therapy," was coined to label the conscious attempt to provide an environment that minimizes pathological behavior such as assault and maximizes clinical progress.[67]

Milieu therapy includes the notion of the therapeutic community and includes psychodynamic, psychological, and behavioral approaches.[68]

In addition to structuring the environment, milieu therapy attempts to structure the patient's schedule so as to provide purposeful activity throughout the day with occupational and recreational therapies.[69]

Such environmental intervention hopefully would minimize irritable, sex related, territorial, predatory, male competitive, maternal and fear induced instrumental aggression in psychiatric facilities.

The doctor has the critical role in the hospital in patient management including management of aggression. The doctor is primarily responsible for the diagnosis and prevention of aggression.

Generally, admission and treatment require a doctor's orders.

The application of physical restraints, medication, ECT and occupational therapy requires a doctor's orders and is within the discretion of the doctor's medical judgment.

Psychiatric diagnosis is currently more art than science. The psychiatric or medical doctor managing a patient must juggle all the imperatives that converge upon the patient.

Although the literature and experience suggest that suicide and homicide (under the rubric of dangerous behavior) are not predictable for the purposes of commitment, the doctor must make a reasonable effort at prediction and management to avoid malpractice ligation and promote the patient's best interest.

Although medications, ECT, and restraints are effective, the doctor must administer them with informed consent or seek judicial intervention. The doctor must provide the least restrictive alternative.[70] The doctor must accept the fact that judicial intervention and conformation to acceptable past practice may not be sufficient to protect him from legal liability.[71]

"Informed" "consent" is a subtle concept with two axis. Each axis allows for opportunity for error.

In an ordinary physician-patient contract, it is difficult to ascertain how much information satisfies "informed" consent.

The doctor has four years of college, four years

of medical school, a year's internship and sometimes three or four years of specialty training in a residency program or fellowship.

Within a matter of minutes or an hour, the doctor examines the patient, makes a diagnosis and recommends treatment. It is highly unlikely that the patient's grasp of the consequences of a given diagnosis or treatment regimen approaches that of the doctor.

In the urgency of an assault or the time constraints of a busy emergency room what constitutes consent? A struggling patient in the hands of four attendants or leather restraints is hardly consenting to i.v. Haldol or ECT. Yet these may be lifesaving procedures in the case of an excited catatonic schizophrenic patient.

Medical malpractice emerges in Michigan only after a duty is established by the creation of the physician-patient relationship.[72]

A doctor may not impose the doctor-patient relationship.[73]

After the doctor-patient contract is established, the physician is not required to guarantee the results, although he is required to exercise the skill, care, knowledge and attention ordinarily possessed and applied by others in similar circumstances.[74]

However, a doctor is free to contract and may or may not warrant the results and may do so as part of the original contract or a separate contract.[75]

After the contract is established, the doctor patient relationship lasts until ended by mutual agreement, revoked by the patient dismissing the doctor or the physician determines his services are no longer useful to the patient and he provides the patient reasonable time to procure alternative medical care.[76]

In Michigan the standard of care is described as thorough and diligent examination and treatment according to the circumstances.[77]

Liability is not measured by the actual methods employed in the community, but by what is recognized as good practice when given a choice of good practices.[79] The standard of care for the specialist in Michigan is the national standard of care according to the school of medicine of the specialist.[80]

The physician's best judgment is sufficient in an emergency.[81]

Informed consent has generated sensational publicity in the breach.[82]

The issues vary according to the circumstances.

Commitment and treatment in the state hospital require a determination of dangerousness by a physician and authorization of treatment by a probate judge in Michigan. The procedures are codified by the Michigan Mental Health Code[83] and regulations filed by the Michigan Department of Mental Health with the Secretary of State.

The use of seclusion and physical restraint are more likely to be utilized than i.v. Haldol or ECT.[84]

In Michigan the quiet room, seclusion, short term physical restraints, drug restraints and other physical restraints are given preference in the order given, i.e. the quiet room most preferred and other physical restraint such as ECT least preferred.

In hospitals, other than state hospitals, it is uncommon to have committed patients.
In private hospitals, patients are generally competent.[85]

There is no presumption in Michigan that a voluntary psychiatric patient cannot refuse treatment or sign out against medical advice.

Some authorities have suggested that incompetence is a condition preceding commitment[86] which would imply that every voluntary patient is competent.

Judicial encroachment upon psychiatric activity has resulted in some extremely interesting results. The right of a quadriplegic to refuse treatment has been tested in the context of "dangerousness" of the quadriplegic patient.[87] Applications of judicial decisions originating in state hospital cases to private hospitals have resulted in heavy fiscal expenditures. "The cases described by the author resulted in expenditures of more than $30,000 by the patients and their insurers."[88]

The physician must evaluate the patient, make a diagnosis, formulate a treatment plan, inform the patient, and obtain consent from the patient or probate court.

His task is not then complete. He must then decide whether he should inform potential victims of the homicidal patient.[89]

If the potential victim already knows, the warning is probably not neessary.[90]

Where the victim provokes the patient into assault there is the possibility of waiver by assumption of the risk.[91]

However, on a psychiatric unit, the provocative behavior may be a product of another patient's mental illness and not voluntary or intentional, so the psychiatrist may retain a duty to warn the victim, the staff, or other physicians to mitigate the liability by providing more distance between the incompatible patients.

A duty to warn may exist only when specific threats to assault a specific individual are made.

However, in a closed environment of a mental health unit of thirty patients plus staff, a general threat may be contained within the specific environment and be specific enough to attach a duty to warn or intervene in some manner. The doctor and hospital do have a special fiduciary responsibility to patient and visitors that they might not have to the public at large.[93]

The physician must evaluate the patient, make a diagnosis, formulate a treatment plan, inform the patient, obtain consent, and warn potential victims and make provisions to protect other patients.

All of this occurs during ordinary practice.

What extraordinary intervening variables may intrude on the physician's routine practices? The most alarming are uncommon but possibly fatal medication side effects or reactions.

Diazepam (Valium), a commonly used medication, is a good example.

Although this drug is useful for interrupting seizures and reducing anxiety, it may produce hyperexcited states, anxiety, hallucinations, increased muscle spasticity, insomnia, rage, sleep disturbances, and stimulation.

The majority of major and minor tranquilizers and antidepressants are capable of producing these paradoxical states. A review of the psychotropic medications and their side effects is easily accomplished by reading the Physician's Desk Reference.[95]

A case of filicide has been reported as a consequence of exposure to psychotropic medication.[96]

The physician must decide how much risk he will assume. The most common strategy is to assess which choice will result in the least mortality and morbidity and advocate that choice. Generally, the use of tranquilizers results in less agitation, and less assault, and less risk as paradoxical excitement is the uncommon exception to the rule of sedation.

Another dilemma is the physician's use of the medical literature.

Anecdotal reports of single cases or small series of cases which do not reach statistical significance are relatively common.

They often promise relief to many without the blessing of official approval. "The authors successfully treated four patients who had irreversible aggressiveness and outbursts of rage, which had not been affected by high doses of major tranquilizers or anticonvulsants."[97]

What risks does the attending physician assume by using or not using propranolol to control rage? Even the use of more accepted medication such as haloperidol is associated with considerable risks that expose the physician to litigation for bad results with good intent. "The rapid neuroleptization (Titration) technique is a method of administering repeat doses of neuroleptic medication under close medical supervision that provides control of acute functional psychotic symptoms in most patients.

The technique is an important landmark because agitated and belligerent patients are often seen clinically. Rapid symptom control not only relieves distressing symptoms, but greatly reduces the risk of injury to self and others."[98]

The use of novel, uncommon or experimental treatments requires separate consideration. A physician is liable for malpractice when it is shown his breach of contract is due to the application of practices that depart from the community standard and results in damage.[99]

However, a physician who treats a patient who has failed to respond to customary care at the hand of other physicians is not guilty of malpractice for trying insufficiently a new treatment, uncommon, but known to achieve good results, where the alternative is amputation.[100] However, such experiments require knowledge and consent by the patient.[101]

After having diagnosed the patient and attending to peripheral matters, the doctor must assess his own position in the "ecological system."

As a forensic psychiatrist, the responsibility is to the state and not the patient. The transaction between the psychiatrist and the patient may be adversary and not medical.[102] The psychiatrist in the commitment procedure and the certifying physician act as officers of the court and not as the patient's agent or independent contractor. Their duties in Michigan are codified by the Mental Health Code.[103]

Often psychiatrists in institutional settings, although identified as being responsible for the welfare of the patients, by virtue of employment by third parties or other coercions are "captured" by the institutions and actually serve the institution's needs first.[104] As a result a "continuing variance between psychiatry's ethical percepts and the practice in such institutions creates an undesirable situation"[105] whereby more and more often, institutional psychiatrists are forced into these practices by the politics and economics of the delivery system."[106]

In Michigan, case law has defined the responsibilities of physicians and psychiatrists employed by third parties. A certifying physician is an officer of the court operating under color of state law and is not liable for assault and battery for commitment."[107]

However, treatment may be given only with consent of the patient except to the extent necessary to prevent injury to the patient or others and at the peril of the superintendant.[108]

Finally, a probate order to detain a person in a private hospital does not mandate treatment or give an implied duty to provide psychiatric treatment.[109]

Examination for third parties for reasons other than diagnosis and treatment for the benefit of the patient will not create liability for malpractice.[110]

Although the psychiatrist and physician contracts to diagnose and treat the patient, warn third parties, and anticipate rare complications, he retains the privilege of protecting himself. Potential assaults are difficult to predict and there are recent reports of homicides in hospital emergency rooms.[111] Some physicians reportedly are responding by carrying guns. Research suggests that approximately 1.9% of patients threaten their therapist and 0.63% of these same patients assault their therapists.[112]

About 24% of a group of 101 therapists studied reported that they themselves had suffered assaults. [113] Some authority advocates martial arts training in unarmed combat for the purpose of minimizing staff and patient injury while subduing violent patients.[114] This is particularly true of urban emergency rooms where many of the psychiatric patients are armed with blunt and sharp weapons and even the occasional gun.[115] At this point the role of the doctor ends and the hospital and police authority begins. At times legal intervention would be more appropriate than medical intervention.[116]

Hospitals have been sheltered by sovereign and charitable immunity in the past. The notion that their activities were independent of medical treatment delivered by physicians further insulated hospitals from malpractice litigation. Recent erosion of these defenses to liability has resulted in rapid changes in hospital policy and procedures to accommodate the new levels of accountability and liability that statutory and case law are evolving. "As a separate legal entity, a hospital is subject to liability under virtually all of the principles of civil and criminal law. The hospital's legal responsibility for the physical and emotional wellbeing of others...typically arises under negligence law, although it can also flow from theories of contract law, express or implied warranty, or strict liability."[117]

This liability may arise from breach of duty established by community standards, hospital rules and by-laws, violation of statutes, res ipse loquitor and contributory or comparative negligence.[118]

The authors point out negligent supervision of patients and protecting the mentally ill as high-risk areas.[119]

In addition, by application of corporate liability theories, hospitals now find themselves liable for acts performed by medical staff, employees, nurses and borrowed servants.[120]

All this potential liability may spring from an assault by a patient in the hospital. This assault may occur in the emergency room; the intensive care unit; coronary care unit; pediatric unit; dialysis unit; diagnostic centers such as cardiology, and cardiopulmonary or on diagnostic leave to other hospital laboratories; and ancillary therapeutic centers such alcohol therapy or physical therapy.

Each of these locations has its own particular problems in patient management.

Add to this complex is the fact that the assault may be a product of "normal" behavior, criminal behavior, or mental illness as previously described. Finally, the assault may be a product of predatory, territorial, fear induced, male competitive, sex-related, irritable, maternal, or instrumental behavior.

What level of conduct must the hospital maintain to reduce assault and avoid liability for negligence? What interventions are available?

The hospital may provide an overwhelming number of employees to intervene in a given assault.[121]

The hospital may provide training in martial

arts skills so that patients may be subdued with the minimum number of injuries.[122]

The hospital may provide quiet rooms, seclusion rooms, physical restraints, and chemical restraints and other physical restraints[123] for the protection of staff when "essential in order to prevent the resident from physically harming himself or others, or in order to prevent substantial property damage."[124]

"The governing body shall establish policies and procedures which define the use of physical restraint and seclusion and which designate who may ignore temporary physical restraint and seclusion."[125]

"The type of physical restraint or condition of seclusion and the duration of the restraint or seclusion and of the clothing to be removed, if any, shall be specified in the order and shall be documented in the residents medical record and further, a record of restraint and seclusion shall be available for inspection by the department of Mental Health at all (mental health facilities using restraint and seclusion and)....a separate, permanent chronological record shall be kept for the purpose of listing specific instances of use of physical restraint or seclusion and shall include all of the following:

(a) The name, age, and sex of the resident.

(b) The type of physical restraint or conditions of seclusion.

(c) Full justification for each application of physical restraint or seclusion, including why the measure is essential and why a less restrictive measure would not suffice.

(d) The name of the authorizing and ordering physician or qualified professional person.

(e) The name of person instituting temporary restraint or seclusion.

(f) The date and time placed in temporary restraint or seclusion.

(g) The date and time removed from temporary, authorized, and ordered physical restraint or seclusion.

(h) A notation of steps taken during the period of physical restraint or seclusion, with regard to examination, opportunities for free movement, food, sanitary conditions, clothing, or other cover, an opportunity to sit or lie down, toilet access, bathing, and telephone calls made on behalf of a resident in seclusion or restraint."[127]

At this time the Department of Mental Health has laid down meticulous guidelines for the management of the assaultive patient. It should be easy by compliance to avoid negligence litigation.

It is more difficult to address the potentially violent patient.

Predatory behavior such as cannibalism may be dealt with by feeding or overfeeding the patient population.

Sex-related aggression may be minimized by segregation or chaperoning patients, providing passes or conjugal visits to dissipate sex drives and by requiring conservative clothing and activities to minimize stimulations.

Territorial aggression may be minimized by providing adequate space and not allowing for overcrowding.

Male competitive aggression may be reduced by providing cooperative activity and a cooperative milieu atmosphere. It may further be dissipated by identifying it on a conscious level and sublimating the energy or interrupting its display with therapeutic contracts or truces.

Maternal aggression is prevented by having a policy of overtly and covertly discouraging critical or hostile exchanges among patients and identifying the emergence of competitive groups or cliques.

Fear induced aggression may be dissipated by adequate medication and reassurance.

Irritable aggression may be disrupted by sublimation or socialization, medication and reducing the frequency of provoking contacts.

Most of these solutions or preventative measures require surveillance and therapeutic interventions.

Where sleeping quarters are shared, it requires judicious room assignments with close observation of interaction. It is uncommon for an assault to erupt without warning signals.

State hospitals must take dangerous patients who are committed.[128]

Other hospitals "may" admit patients by application and certificate. Hospitals are generally reluctant to accept dangerous patients, even voluntary patients.

"June 15, 1982
Dear Doctor (redacted)
Mr. L... has shared with me a letter from you regarding the need for general and acute homicidal precautions in this hospital. Please be advised that the hospital is not equipped or prepared to handle homicidal patients. Such patients, if known, should not be admitted to this facility. If a patient is admitted and found to be homicidal, that patient must be transferred, at the earliest moment, to an institution having facilities to handle this type of patient. Such action only supports our care and concern for the other patients in the Mental Health Unit.
Yours truly,
(signature redacted)
Administrator

This letter and its tone are subject to the following criticisms.

First, given the ubiquity of aggression in our

culture it is not possible to design a screening procedure that will prevent the admission of homicidal patients.

Psychiatrists are not able to predict dangerousness. Indeed, psychiatrists are not able to save their own lives from assault by patients. As a result, homicidal precautions are necessary even on a unit that has a policy of transferring psychiatric patients to other facilities.

Second, to the small degree that assault is predictable, training in homicidal precautions will facilitate identification and intervention whether or not transfer is hospital policy as part of the intervention.

Third, if another facility is capable of managing dangerous patients, how may any facility justify not sharing that expertise.[129] It is conceded that it is hard work to manage aggressive patients, "A potentially violent or destructive patient on an inpatient service often provokes strained communication patterns in both patient and staff."[130] However, from a behavior perspective, "when he general hospital psychiatric inpatient unit is unwilling to accept the involuntarily hospitalized patient, is unwilling in many cases to accept the indigent patient, feels incapable of managing the disruptive, aggressive, or acutely suicidal patient....it is failing to serve the psychiatric needs of an appreciable segment of the community,...."[131]

The Michigan Mental Health Code requires a suitable, safe, sanitary and humane environment.[132] Even if the facility were to have a policy of identifying and removing homicidal patients, for the period of time necessary to arrange discharge and transfer homicidal precautions would probably be necessary for the safety of patients and staff.

At this time, the "major social process affecting general hospital psychiatry today (is) deinstitutionalization."[133] The result is that the general hospital will receive the same patients back from the community that it is transferring to the state hospital as "homicidal." Such an exercise in futility serves little purpose. This trend is not likely to change. It is a product of state fiscal policies and legislative and judicial action asserting patients' rights to treatment and the least restrictive surroundings.[134]

A final consideration is the result of rejecting an aggressive patient. There is much research on the efficacy of psychiatric treatment. It is easy to doubt the effect of such an intangible as psychiatric intervention. The concrete changes of surgery are not available. The objective measures available to internal medicine are not available. "No doubt, practitioners of psychotherapy find the lack of research support for its effectiveness disheartening."[135] With this and a reluctance to accept the work and responsibility of an aggressive patient, it is easy to justify administrative discharge. However, there is evidence that some patients do suffer from irregular discharges from hospitals.[136]

It may eventually be shown that all patients irregularly discharged suffer actual harm. Intuitively, it seems to be quite a loss to lose hope of improvement to the point that hospitalization is not allowed or considered worthwhile.

Michigan case law originally recognized the distinctions between private for profit hospitals[137], charitable hospitals[138] and state hospitals.[139] The standard of care of the private hospital for its administrators and employees is reasonable care and attention. The nature of such attention is determined by the circumstances.[140] The standard of care for a nurse's aide assisting an elderly patient to the bathroom is that of an ordinary and careful prudent person under similar circumstances.[141] A surgeon does not become an agent of the hospital simply by using the hospital facilities.[142]

The charitable immunity defense in Michigan was overruled by judicial decisions.[143] Where circumstances permit an inference of hospital negligence, the hospital must come forward with an explanation for the cause of the injury.[144] However, where the hospital provides facilities for the public according to state statute, the agency may be entitled to statutory immunity under Mich. Comp. Laws Section 691.1407.[145] The issue turns upon whether the hospital is performing a governmental function as opposed to a proprietary function.[146] In the context of assault by patients, application of restraints and other interventions are arguably an exercise of the state police power or parens patriae sufficient to cloak even a private hospital under the protection of governmental immunity. The rule removing the defense of governmental immunity from municipally owned hospitals is properly applied to any case pending on December 27, 1978 or starting after that time.[147] The test is whether the hospital services could be delivered by other than governmental hospitals.[148] Finally, a hospital may be held liable on the theory of respondent superior for the acts of agents and employees including malpractice.[149]

Michigan still recognizes the defense of sovereign immunity for state hospitals.[150] Hospital's liability for injury as a result of application of restraints has been contested outside of Michigan.[151]

A hospital's liability for injury or death of a doctor, nurse or attendant has also been given consideration.[152]

Liability for an assault by a patient by another patient has been argued as early as 1907.[153] "They knew a person so affected might reasonably be expected to become violent, uncontrollable, and dangerous at anytime, they should have taken such reasonable precautions with reference to his control or confinement as would have prevented his inflicting injury upon other inmates of the hospital, that nevertheless, this powerful man, crazed from the excessive use of spiritous liquors, and by reason of that fact uncontrollable and dangerous, was left in an insecure apartment and in charge of a lone woman, who was utterly powerless to restrain him; that under those circumstances, it would seem to a reasonable mind that what happened was to have been expected, if not inevitable; that there was, therefore, some evidence of negligence to go to the jury; and that, in the light of that evidence, the verdict finding the defendant guilty of negligence could not be found unauthorized,"[154]

Recent Supreme Court decisions have applied federal law to assaults by patients in hospitals and the use of various interventions to control assaults. The state must: provide for reasonable personal safety; provide for freedom from undue restraint (the least restrictive alternative); and provide minimal adequate treatment to assure safety and avoid undue restraint. Liability for violation of these imperatives, even in the presence of a compelling state interest, is measured according to professional judgment under the

14th Amendment.[155]

Assault by patients in hospitals result in potential liability for the doctor and the hospital. The doctor must apply professional judgment in assessing potential assaultive behavior, ordering treatment and restraint, and warning potential victims and hospital staff. The specialist is measured by a national standard while the general practitioner is measured by the local standard. While treating the voluntary patient, the doctor operates under the principles of contract law and informed consent. While providing medical certification, the doctor functions as an officer of the court and has the protection of governmental immunity,

The hospital may be a private, a municipal or a state hospital. The private hospital has liability according to theories of contract, respondeat superior and corporate liability for actions of its officers and agents for tortious acts of negligence and malpractice. Charitable immunity is not available as a defense for torts in Michigan. Governmental immunity is not available to municipal hospitals. The distinction between proprietary functions and governmental functions probably remains viable as a source of protection from common law tort in Michigan. However, federal law provides potential for liability and legal relief for injury arising from commitment procedures for those acts violating due process and equal protection under the 14th Amendment.

The trend is for continuously greater accountability for doctors and hospitals in their management of patients.

The declarative notion that the sovereign can do no wrong is becoming the notion that the Sovereign can do no harm as the imperative command of the people.

The notion that charities ought to be forgiven for error has changed to the notion that it is unbecoming and unforgivable that a charity be negligent.

Doctors and hospitals are being held to higher standards. Intuitively, it seems appropriate that doctors and hospitals be treated as fiduciaries. They hold themselves out as skilled, licensed, and professional. They cannot function without the trust of the patient and the community. Any relationship grounded upon trust must be characterized as a fiduciary relationship, whether parent, pastor, doctor, hospital or political office. Any accountability other than a fiduciary accountability invites abuse and neglect. The treatment of the patient ought to be based upon the patient's best interest and not the convenience or personal interest of the doctor or hospital.

1.   C. M. Bell M.D., J. Palmer M.A., <u>Security Procedures in a Psychiatric Emergency Service</u> 73:9 Journal of the National Medical Association 835 (1981).
2.   Kaimowitz v. Department of Mental Health for the State of Michigan Circuit Court for the County of Wayne, Michigan, July 10, 1973. Civil Action No. 73-19434-AW <u>Law and Bioethics 291 (1982),</u> T. Shannon, J. Manfra.
3.   Administrative Rules, Michigan Department of Mental Health, filed with the Secretary of State on December 11, 1981 (Available for $3.50 by writing the Department of Mental Health, Office Services, Sixth Floor, Lewis Cass Building, Lansing, Michigan 48926
4.   Letter
"June 15, 1982
Dear Doctor (redacted)

Mr. L... has shared with me a letter from you regarding the need for general and acute homicidal precautions in this hospital. Please be advised that the hospital is not equipped or prepared to handle homicidal patients. Such patients, if known, should not be admitted to this facility. If a patient is admitted and found to be homicidal, that patient must be transferred, at the earliest moment, to an institution having facilities to handle this type of patient. Such action only supports our care and concern for the other patients in the Mental Health Unit.

   Yours truly,
   (signature redacted)
   Administrator

5. L. Weinreb, Criminal Law 3 (1980) ("it is not always a crime to kill someone intentionally...") P. Corining, Ph.d., "Collective Aggression," Comprehensive Textbook of Psychiatry I 316 (1975)

6. L. Weinreb, supra note 5 at 203 C. Corning, B.A., P Corning "Aggressive behavior," Comprehensive Book of Psychiatry II 310 (1975) (hereinafter cited as psychological aggression)

7. L. Weinreb, supra note 5 at 353 (Cited as The Queen v. Dudley and Steavens, 14 Q.B.

273 (----35) All B.R. Rep. 61 (1884). A crew stranded at seas in a live boat out of desperation killed and ae a cabin boy. Two members were convicted and sentenced to six months in jail. C. Corning and P. Corning supra note 6 at 311

8. L. Weinreb, supra note 5 at 204 C. Corning and P. Corning supra note 6 at 311.

9. L. Weinreb, supra note 5 at 65 C. Corning and P. Corning supra note 6 at 311

10. L. Weinreb, supra note 5 at 231 et. Seq. C. Corning and P. Corning supra
 note 6 at 312

11. L. Weinreb, supra note 5 at 222 C. Corning and P. Corning supra note 6 at 312

12. L. Weinreb, supra note 5 at 68 C. Corning and P. Corning supra note 6 at 312

13. L. Weinreb, supra note 5 at 66 C. Corning and P. Corning supra note 6 at 312

14. L. Weinreb, supra note 5 at 570 et. seq. C. Corning and P. Corning supra
 note 6 at 312

15. P. Hollinger, M.D., M.P.H., "Violent Death as a Leading Cause of Mortality: An Epidemiologic Study of Suicide, Homicide, and Accident," 139:8 AM. J. Psych. 1028 (Aug 1982)

16. Id.

17. S. Gerson, Ph.D. E. Bassuk, M.D., "Psychiatric Emergencies: An Overview" .137:1 Am. J. Psych. 1 (Jan. 1980)
18. Id.
19. R. Schwiczgebel, "Prediction of Aggressiveness and its Implications for Treatment," Modern Legal Medicine, Psychiatry and Forensic Science 734 (1980)
20. Id, at 785
21. Id, at 785
22. Id, at 785
23. Id, at 785
24. Id, at 785
25. T. Craig, "An Epidemiological Study of Problems Associated with Violence Among Psychiatric Patients," 139:10 Am. J. Psych. 1265 (Oct. 1982).
26. J. Simonds and J. Kashani, "Drug Abuse and Criminal Behavior in Delinquent Boys Committed to a Training School," 136:11 Am. J. Pscyh 1444 1444 (Nov. 1979.)
27. N. Fauman, M.D., Ph.D. and B. Bauman, M.D., "Violence Associated with Phencyclidine Abuse," 136:12 Am. J. Psych. 1584 (Dec. 1979).
28. D. Lewis, M.D., J. Pincus, M.D., E. Shanon, M.P.H., and G. Glasser, M.D., "Psychomotor Epilepsy and Violence in a Group of Incarcerated Adolescent Boys," 137:7 Am. J.

Psych. 882 (July 1982.)

29. S. Mednick, M.D., "Biology's 'role' in Crime May Lead to Changes in Law," Psychiatric News Vol W/III No. 18 9 (Sept. 17, 1982

30. G. Rogeness, M.D., J. Hernandez, M.D., S. Nacelo, M.D., and E. Mitchell, M.D. "Biochemical Differences in Children with Conduct Disorder Socialized and Undersocialized," 139:3 Am. J. Psych, 307,310 (March 1982). (Low DBH in Plasma of Undersocialized Children)

31. C. Brown, M.D., M Eibert, M.D., I. Moyon, M.D., D. Jimerson, M.D., W. Kilein M.D., W. Bunnez, M.D., F Goodwin M.D., "Aggression, Suicide and Serotonin: Relationships to CSF Amine Metabolites," 139:6 Am. J. Psych. (June 1982).

32. T. Craig, Supra Note 25

33. L. Weinreb, supra Note 5 at 293

34. L. Weinreb, supra Note 5 at 1 et. Seq. (The Problem of Definition)

35. L. Weinreb, supra Note 5 at 432-518

36. L. Weinreb, supra Note 5 at 481

37. S. Divitz, Ph.D., "The Antisocial Personality," Modern Legal Medicine Psychiatry and Forensic Science 779 (1980)

38. L. Weinreb, supra Note 5 at 696 et. Seq. (recidivist statutes).
39. S. Dinitz Ph.D., supra note 37 at 906
40. Id
41. H. Roth, M.P.H., "Correctional Psychiatry," Modern Legal Medicine Psychiatry and Forensic Science, 677, 7000 (1980)
42. Id. at 688
43. J.C., Ph.D., and J. J. Bonovitz M.D., "Diversion of the Mentally Ill Into the Criminal Justice System: The Police Intervention Perspective," 318:7 Am. J. Psych. 973 (July 1981)
44. D. Lewis, M.D., J. Pincuk, M.D., S. Shanok, M.P.H., and G. Gilbert, M.D., "Psychomotor Epilepsy and Violence in a Group of Incarcerated Adolescent Boys," 139:7 Am. J. Psych. 882 (July 1982)
45. J. Simons, M.D., J. Kashani, M.D., "Drug Abuse and Criminal Behavior in Delinquent Boys Committed to a Training School," 136:11 Am. J. Psych. 1449 (Nov. 1979) (Amphetamines, Alcohol).
46. R. Pasawask, Ph.D., M. Pantle, M.A., and R. Steadman, Ph.D., "Detention and Rearrest Rates of Persons Found Guilty By Reason of Insanity, and Convicted Felons." 139:7 Am. J. Psych. 892 (July 1982).

47. S. Inandar, M.D., D. Lewis, M.D., G Giomopoulos, M.D., S. Shanok, M.P.H., amella, M.D., "Violent and Suicidal Behavior in Psychotic Adolescents," 139:7 Am. J. Psych. 932 (July 1982).
48. T. Hackett, "The Disruptive State," The Massachusetts General Hospital Handbook of General Psychiatry, 246 (1978)
49. Id.
50. Id.
51. G. Murray, "Confusion, Delirium, and Dementia," The Massachusetts General Hospital Handbook of General Psychiatry, 93, 112 (1978)
52. Medical Economics Company, Physician's Desk Reference, 1158 et seq. (1982)
53. Id.
54. L. Linn, "Other Psychiatric Emergencies," 2 Comprehensive Textbook of Psychiatry/II, 1785, 1787 (1975)
55. Id.
56. Id.
57. Id.
58. Id.
59. Id. at 1787, 88.
60. R. Schwictzgebel, "Prediction of Dangerousness and Its Implication for Treatment," Modern Legal Medicine Psychiatry

Forensic Science," 783, 788 (1980).

61. C. Wilkinson and W. O'Connor, "Human Ecology and Mental Illness," 139:8 Am. J. Psych. 985 (August 1982)
62. Id.
63. R. Goodstein and A. Page, "Battered Wife-Syndrome: Overview of Dynamics and Treatment," 138:8 Am. J. Psych. 1036 (1981)
64. M. Wolfgang, "Suicide by Means of Victim Mediated Homicide, 20 J. of Clinical Experimental Psychopathology 335-349 (1959). L. Selter and C. Payne "Automobile Accidents, Suicide and Unconscious Motivation," 119 Am. J. Psych. 237-240 (1962). C. Hollinger, "Violent Death as a Leading Cause of Mortality: An Epidemiologic Study of Psychiatry of Suicide, Homicide and Accident," 137:4 Am. J. Psych. 472 (April 1980)
65. L. Linn, "Other Psychiatric Emergencies," 2 Comprehensive Textbook of Psychiatry II, 1785, 1787 (1975)
66. Id.
67. A. Freedman, H. Kaplan, B. Sadock, "Chapter 32 Milieu Therapy," Comprehensive Textbook of Psychiatry II 1990-2009 (1975)
68. Id. at 1994

69. L. Lynn, "Occupational Therapy and Other Therapeutic Activities" 2 Comprehensive Textbook of Psychiatry II 2003 (1975)

70. Smith v. Michigan, Mich. Ct. Cl. Bc 79-6758 (Jan. 29, 1981).

Youngberg v. Romeo 50 LW 4681 (June 15 1982)

P. Appelbaum and T. Gutheil, "The Boston State Hospital Case: 'Involuntary Mind Control,' and the Right to Rot," 137:6 Am. J. Psych," 718 (June 1980)

71. O'Connor v. Donaldson 422 US 563 (1975).
72. Parker v. Sables 79 Mich. App. 386 (1977)
73. Stowers v. Wolodzko 19 Mich. App, 115 (1969)
74. Viland v. Wilson 34 Mich. App 485 (1971)
    Sheffington v. Bradley 366 Mich 556 (1962).
75. Guilmet v. Campbell 385 Mich. 57 (1971)
76. Fortner v. Koch 272 Mich. 273 (1935)
77. Rostron v. Klein 23 Mich. App. 288 (1976).
78. Burton v. Smith 34 Mich. App. 270 (1971)
79. Rytkones v Lojacondo 269 Mich. 270 (1934)
80. Ferguson v. Gonyan 64 Mich. App. 685 (1975)
81. Rostron v. Klein 23 Mich. App. 288 (1976).
82. Kaimowitz v Department of Mental Health for the State of Michigan, Circuit

Court for the County of Wayne, Michigan, July 10, 1973 Civil Action
No 73, -19434-AW, Reproduced in T. Shannon and J. Manfra,
Law and Bioethics 200 (1982)

83. Mich. Comp. Laws 330.1423 et. seq.
84. Mich. Comp. Laws 330.1716 Consent.
    330.118   Chemotherapy
    330.1740   Physical Restraints.
    330.1741   Seclusion
    R330.7243 Restraint and Seclusion, Administrative Rules of the Michigan Department of Mental Health Filed Deccember 11, 1981.
85. Mich. Comp. Laws Section 330.1702 Rights and Competency not affected by receipt of services, determiknations, or admission to a facility,
86. B. Labeque and L. Clark, "Incompetence to Refuse Treatment: A Necessary Condition for Civil Commitment," 138:8 Am. J. Psych. 1076 (August 1981)
87. R. Part and D. Turns, "Dangerousness and the Right of a Psychotic Quadraplegic Patient to Refuse Treatment," 137:5 Am. J. Psych. 623 (May 1980).
88. I. Ferr, Éffect of the Rennie Decision on Private Hospitalization in New Jersey: Two

Case Reports, 138:6 <u>Am. J. Psych</u> 774 (June 1981).
89. Tarasoff v. Regents of the University of California, 551 P.2d 334 (1976).
D. Kjervik, "The Psychiatric Nurse's Duty to Warn Potential Victions of Homicidal Psychotherapy Outpatients," 9:6 <u>Law, Medicine and Healthcare</u> 11 (Dec. 1981)
90. Hawkins v. County Department of Rehabilitative Services, 602 P. 2d. 361 (1979)
91. Leedy v. Harnett, 510 F. Supp. 1125, 1131 (1981).
92. Thompson v. County of Alamada 614 F. 2d. 728 (1980).
93. Id.
94. Medical Services Co. Physicians Desk Reference, 1625 (1982)
95. Id.
96. D. Luchins et. al., "Filicide During Drug-Induced Somnambulism: A <u>Case</u> Report," 135:11 <u>Am. J. Psych</u> 1404 (N D. ov. 1978).
97. S. Yudofsky, D. Williams, J. Gorman, "Propranolol in the Treatment of Rage and Violent Behavior in Patients with Chronic Brain Syndromes," 138:2 <u>Am. J. Psych</u>. 218 (February 1981).
98. P. Donlon, J. Hopkin, J. Tupin, "Overview: Efficacy and Safety of the Rapid

Neuroleptization Method with Injectable Haloperidol," 136:3 Am. J. Psych. 273 (March 1979)

99. McPhee v Bay City Samaritan Hospital 10 Mich. App. 517 (1968) Id, at 785

100. Miller v. Tolen 183 Mich. 252 (1914)

101. Portner v. Kock 272 M 273 (1935)

102. J. Rappaport, "Differences Between Forensic and General Psychiatry," 139:9 Am. J. Psych. 331 (March 1982).

103. Mich. Comp. Laws 330.1423 et. seq. Mich. Department of Mental Health R330.7243 Restraint and Seclusion," Administrative Rules 116 Filed with Secretary of State (Dec. 11, 1981).

104. Supra note 25.

105. B. Burnstein, " 'Medical Responsibility' in Institutional Settings,"
137:9 Am. J. Psych, 1071 (September 1980)

106. Id. at 1073

107. Stowers v. Wolodzko 386 Mich. 119 (1981)

108. Stowers v. Wolodzko 386 Mich. 119 (1981)
Olepa v. Mapletoff 2 Mich. App. 734 (1966)

109. Id.

110. Rogers v. Horvath 65 Mich. App, 644 (1975)

111. H. McCann, "Packin Iron," 110th Year no.

45 Detroit News 1 October 6, 1982
- 112. C. Bell and J. Palmer, "Security Procedures in a Psychiatric Emergency Service," Vol. 73, No 9 J. of the National Medical Association 835 (1981)
- 113. Id.
- 114. Id.
- 115. Id.
- 116. T. Craig, "An Epidemiological Study of Problems Associated with Violence Among Psychiatric Patients," 139:10 Am. J. Psych. 1262,1265 (October 1982)
- 117. Aspen Systems Corporation Health Law Center, Principles of Hospital Liability," Law Manual 1 et seq (1980)
- 118. Id. Sections 2-1 through 2-5.
- 119. Id. Sections 3-5 and 3-6.
- 120. Id. Sections 4-1 through 4-4.
- 121. C. Bell supra at note 4
  T. Hackett supra at note 1.
  L. Linn supra at note 7.
- 122. C. Bell supra at note 48
- 123. Mich. Department of Mental Health R330.7243 Restraint and Seclusion," Administrative Rules 116 Filed with Secretary of State (Dec. 11, 1981).

124. Mich. Comp. Laws 330.1740 (2)
　　　Restraints 330.1742 (2)
　　　Seclusion 330.1740 (2)
125. Mich. Department of Mental <u>Health</u> <u>supra</u>, note 59 at 117 R 330.7243
　　　Rule 7243 (4)
126. Id. at 117 Rule 7243 (7) (6)
127. Id. at 117 Rule 7243 (5)
128. Mich. Comp. Laws 330.1423
　　　Hospitalization pending certification by psychiatrist:
　　　Application and physician's certificate; Designation of Hospitals.
　　　Sec. 423 A hospital designated by the department shall, and any hospital may, hospitalize an individual presented to the hospital, pending certification for hospitalization by a psychiatrist, if an application and physician's certificate for hospitalization of the individual have been executed. The Department shall designate those department hospitals that are required to hospitalize individuals pursuant to this section,
129. L. Bachrach, "General Hospital Psychiatry: Overview from a Sociological

Perspective," 138:7 Am. J. Psych, 879, 883 (July 1981) "In fact, Becker wrote that 'the involuntarily committed patient can be treated within the general hospital without disruption of the therapeutic milieu."

130. R. Cornfield and S. Fielding, "Impact of the Threatening Patient on Ward Communications," 137:5 Am. J. Psych, 616 (May 1980).
131. L. Bachrach supra note 65 at 883.
132. Mich. Comp. Laws Section 330.1708
133. L. Bachrach supra note 65 at 881.
134. P. Braun et al, "Overview: Deinstitutionalization of Psychiatric Patients.
A Critical Review of Outcome Studies," 138:6 Am. J. Psych.736 (June 1981).8
135. N. Epstein and L. Vlok, "Research on the Results of Psychotherapy:
A Summary of Evidence," 138: Am. J. Psych, 1027, 1033 (August 1981).
136. I. Glick, et. al., "Outcome of Irregularly Discharged Psychiatric Patients," 11 Am. J. Psych. 1472 (November 1981)
137. Rodgers v. Lincoln Hospital 239 Mich.
138. Downes v. Harper Hospital 101 Mich. 555 (1894).

139. Martinson v City of Alpena 328 Mich. 595 (1950)
140. Paulen v. Shinnick 291 Mich. 288 (1939)
141. Fogel v Sinai Hospital of Detroit 2 Mich. App. 99 (1965)
142. Heins v Synkonis 58 Mich. App. 119 (1975)
143. Parker v. Port Huron Hospital 361 Mich. 1 (1960).
144. Hand v. Park Community Hospital 14 Mich. App. 371 (1968).
145. Snow v. Freeman 55 Mich. App. 84 (1974).
146. Lockaby v. County of Wayne 63 Mich. App. 185 (1975).
147. Murray v. Beyer Memorial Hospital 409 Mich. App. 217 (1980).
148. Churchwell v. Board of Regents of University of Michigan,
    97 Mich. App. 463 (1980);
    Pearshall v. Williams 93 Mich. App. 231 (1979)
149. Johnson v. Childrens Hospital 105 Mich. App. 539 (1981).
150. Perry v. Kalamazoo State Hospital, 404 Mich. App. 539 (1981).
151. 25 ALR 3d 1450
152. 1 ALR 3d 1036

153. University of Louisville v Hammock 127 Ky 564, 106 S.W. 219 (1907).
154. W. Habeeb, "Liability of Hospitals for Injury Caused Through Assault by a Patient," 48 A.L.R. 3rd 1288.
155. Youngsberg v. Romeo, 457 U.S. 307; 102 S. Ct. 2452 (1982).

Post Script: Copyright applied for January 6th, 2020 by William Yee, M.D., J.D.

The author's first experience with aggression was at the hands of his grandmother, "Billy, go to the lilac bush and bring me back a switch."

That was in 1952 when I was five. I went to the lilac bush and broke off a switch. I stripped the twigs and leaves from the switch.

I don't recall how or when I learned to do this task.

I brought the switch to my grandmother. She held my hand and switched my calves. I danced around her in a circle because she was holding my hand. To this day I do not recall why she switched me. I do not recall that she was being mean or cruel.

I believe that I did something wrong and she was applying a reasonable corrective action. I have no anger or fear arising from this memory.

Between 1953 and 1958 I recall fights among the children in the trailer park.

The fights had rules. We did not use clubs or knives. We did not strike with fists or attempt to injure our adversary.

We wrestled and gained control.

When the adversary was subdued and helpless, we demanded, "say uncle."

I always wound up saying, "uncle," and I would be humiliated and hung my head low when I looked at my friends when I was freed.

I avoided every fight I could, but when challenged in front of my friends, I would fight, even when I knew I was going to say, "uncle," in front of my friends. Not fighting was more humiliating than saying, "uncle."
In junior high school and high school there were fights with fists, clubs and chains.

I did not participate. Being small was not an advantage I wished to exploit.

When I went to work at the factories in Detroit there were guns, muggings and murders mixed in with the loan sharking, prostitution and drug dealing in the Chrysler factories where worked from 1965 to 1971.

When I attended Wayne State University in Detroit, Michigan from 1966 to 1983 there were murders and rapes of students and faculty members on campus and the nearby apartment buildings that students and graduate students lived in while working and going to school.

I attended Wayne State University from 1966 to 1983 and graduated from medical school in 1972 and I graduated from law school in 1983.

In 1987 I applied for the position of Director of Mental Health Services for the Michigan Department of Corrections. The first interview went well, and I was invited back for a second interview.

I fully expected to be hired for the position at the second interview.

However, when I arrived, the person who was interviewing me was no longer employed by the Michigan Department of Corrections.

The reason the person had been dismissed was he had signed a Compliance Agreement with the United States Attorney General to end practices that resulted in cruel and unusual conditions in the care of the mentally ill among the prisoners in the Michigan Department of Corrections.

In the past three out of four state hospital and state prison systems were under the supervision of federal courts for failure to provide minimal care for the mentally ill prisoner or state hospital patient.

Michigan had one of the state hospital systems under federal supervision. The constitutional standard that triggered the supervision was not the national standard of a specialist or the local standard of the general practitioner, but "shocks the conscience," standard of constitutional law.

The state prisons and state hospitals tended to treat the federal courts as the enemy rather than an agent for positive change.

As a result, I was hired in as a Psychiatrist III providing direct care of prisoners at the Riverside Psychiatric Hospital, Ionia, Michigan.

The Riverside Psychiatric Hospital was a prison psychiatric hospital with razor wire housing the one hundred most violent prisoners in the state of Michigan from 1987 to 1991 when I was there.

Riverside Psychiatric Hospital was a one hundred bed facility with four twenty-five bed units. Two units were on the ground floor and two units were on the second floor.

The wardens of the Michigan Department of Corrections were held accountable for injuries to prisoners and staff.

I was told that the wardens were given the authority to label any violent prisoner as mentally ill and order transfer to the Riverside Psychiatric Hospital.

Riverside Psychiatric hospital had no authority to refuse admission of these patients.

All that Riverside psychiatric hospital could do was discharge a patient to open a bed and admit the new patient.

When the other prisons started getting more violent patients than they sent out they stopped sending patients.

That is how Riverside wound up with the most violent prisoners and 5.4 workman compensation cases per month, time off due to injuries from assaults by prisoners each month.

When I was at Riverside I was treated as the enemy by many correctional officers. When I arrived on the unit, the Sargent would act as the town crier and yell out loudly, "Dr. Yee alert." Everyone was polite to me, but I was regarded as risky to be around.

The warden was a clinical psychologist and I believe that Riverside Psychiatric Hospital was an experiment in controlling violence with mental health interventions.

Because the medications were not effective the psychiatrists used wrist and ankle restraints to control violence. The workman compensation cases went from 5.4 per month to 2.2 per month because the wrist and ankle restraints were more effective than the medications

The courts determined that the wrist and ankle restraints were cruel and unusual, so the psychiatrists switched to one-to-one supervision and the workman compensation rates stayed at 2.2 per month because one to one supervision was more effective than medications.

Riverside psychiatric hospital was closed after I left in 1991. What the Michigan Department of Corrections learned was that restraints were more effective than medications. Restraints in General Population were by order of correctional officers and not by medical order when I returned to Ionia in 2009. This eliminated the Joint Commission and medical regulation of restraints.

Since I left Riverside Psychiatric Hospital in 1991, I have not seen much improvement in care in state hospitals and prisons in Michigan,

Kentucky and California. They tend to remain understaffed. Medical staff continue to be injured at a regular rate. The nurses are at the greatest risk.

A major change in the condition of employment since 1991 is enhancement of laws that bar discrimination.

You cannot discriminate based on age, gender, sexual orientation, religion, height, weight, etc.

I have seen a very cynical application of the laws that bar discrimination. These laws are utilized to force little old grandmothers to manage young, large, violent criminals and mentally ill patients in state hospitals and prisons. It would be discrimination not to allow them employment and an opportunity to manage the violent patients.

This is not a commonsense application of a rule that bars discrimination. It is a cynical application of the law that is abusive to the employees. Managing a young, large, strong violent patient who has trained in martial arts on the streets requires the rules applied to combat sports such as boxing or mixed martial arts in the octagon.

Females are not allowed to fight males in combat sports. They should not be required to manage violent male patients in prisons and state hospitals.

Fighters are divided into weight classes so that small men and women are not allowed to fight large men and women. Security should be young, strong males managing violent male patients and young strong females managing violent female patients. This is common sense and not employment discrimination.

Women are not equal to men is sports as is demonstrated when transgender females (biological males) are allowed to compete against biological females in sporting events. The transgender females (biological males) dominate the biological females in sporting events. This is easily found in the news. It is not a surprise.

In a prison and state hospital there should not be any fair fight between staff and patient.

The staff should be equal in size weight and age to the patient or in fact younger, stranger and bigger and better trained in martial arts and should outnumber the patient by three to five to one before the assault.

Security should in fact be separate from nursing, doctoring, arts and crafts, social working, etc.

The show of force should occur before the assault, and not after the assault. Security should be visible on the unit in groups of three to five at all times for the safety of the patients and staff. The assault that doesn't happen is the injury that doesn't happen.

If in fact the patient needs to be treated by the nurse, the patient's arms and legs should be secured before the treatment for the safety of the patient as well as the nurse. This should not be viewed as restraint for violence, but as part of the treatment, as securing the limb reduces injuries while drawing blood and providing other health care interventions.

You say that the patient should not be put into a cage for treatment or chained to a chair for treatment.

There are simple and reasonable alternatives.

If in fact the psychiatrist, social worker and psychologist needs to see the patient one on one for privacy, there can be a cage in the room and the psychiatrist, social worker and psychologist can be in the cage with the computer and other equipment that needs to be safe from destruction by the violent patient.

I have sat alone in a room with more than one patient that has murdered or permanently disabled a former psychiatrist. I was at risk and fully aware of it. The above intervention for my safety was not available. State Hospitals and State Prisons in general are very dangerous places to work. Simple interventions are not applied. Criminal negligence on the part of state agencies who claim governmental immunity, say you?

I suggest that governmental immunity is ripe for challenges on many fronts.

A root cause analysis for every assault and injury should result in a prevention of future injuries by virtue of a systemic intervention or a tailored intervention for a particular violent individual or both.

I suggest that a lack of such a root cause analysis and intervention is sufficient to support a judgment against the chain of command all the way to the state capital.

Individual and class action lawsuits are available in every state.

This book is an introduction to the reader. Medical and Legal Advice is not intended or offered. Medical and Legal Advice should be obtained from a lawyer or doctor retained to examine you and your situation in detail before offering medical and legal advice.

This book offers the vocabulary and fundamental knowledge to assist you in understanding what information to offer your personal attorney and physician and what questions to ask.

William Yee M.D., J.D. Board Certified Psychiatrist practicing psychiatry in Michigan, Indiana, Kentucky, Texas, and California since 1972 without interruption at your service.

"Pre-Existing text," includes names of symptoms and medical illnesses, medications, people, corporations, law cases, statutes, text of statutes, the titles of articles and books, the content of articles and books cited, FDA Labels and FDA releases and images taken from the internet.

My copyright claim is a claim to the "original text," which is my personal experience as described in the text and my commentary on names of symptoms and medical illnesses, medications, people, corporations, law cases, statutes, text of statutes, the titles of articles and books, the content of articles and books cited, FDA Labels and FDA releases and images taken from the internet.

www.ingramcontent.com/pod-product-compliance
Lightning Source LLC
Chambersburg PA
CBHW072237170526
45158CB00002BA/938